FERTILITY RECIPES FOR MEN AND WOMEN

Culinary solutions for enhanced reproductive health

Smith Robertson

COPYRIGHT ©

© [2024] by Smith Robertson

TABLE OF CONTENT

CHAPTER 1

INTRODUCTION

In the pursuit of enhancing fertility, the role of nutrition stands as a crucial cornerstone. This guide aims to navigate the intricate relationship between diet and reproductive health, specifically focusing on "Fertility Recipes for Women." Understanding the impact of food choices on fertility sets the stage for a journey towards well-being.

As we delve into this exploration, the purpose is clear: to provide a comprehensive resource for women seeking to optimize their fertility through mindful and nourishing eating habits. By the end of this guide, you'll not only have insights into the essential nutrients for reproductive health but also a collection of delectable recipes designed to support your fertility journey. Let's embark on this path of nutrition and empowerment for women's reproductive wellness.

BRIEF OVERVIEW OF THE IMPORTANCE OF NUTRITION FOR FERTILITY

Nutrition plays a pivotal role in fertility, acting as a silent architect in the intricate process of conception. The body's reproductive system relies on a delicate balance of vitamins, minerals, and other nutrients to function optimally. Adequate nutrition not only supports hormonal balance but also influences egg and sperm development.

The impact of dietary choices extends beyond the physiological realm, influencing overall health and well-being. A well-nourished body is better equipped to handle the demands of pregnancy and foster a healthy environment for fetal development.

In this context, this guide explores the specific nutrients and foods that contribute to reproductive health, offering a roadmap for individuals aspiring to enhance their fertility through mindful and targeted nutritional choices.

PURPOSE OF THE GUIDE

The primary purpose of this guide is to empower women on their fertility journey by providing actionable insights and practical resources. By focusing on "Fertility Recipes for Women," our aim is to offer a comprehensive resource that goes beyond general advice. This guide strives to:

1. **Educate:** Provide a deeper understanding of the connection between nutrition and fertility, unraveling the science behind dietary choices.

2. **Inspire:** Offer a collection of fertility-friendly recipes that are not only nutritious but also delicious, making the journey towards enhanced fertility enjoyable.

3. **Guide:** Navigate readers through various meals and snacks designed to support reproductive health, with clear instructions and explanations of the nutritional benefits.

4. **Empower:** Equip individuals with the knowledge to make informed dietary decisions, fostering a sense of control and agency in their fertility-enhancing efforts.

Ultimately, this guide aspires to be a trusted companion, offering valuable information and practical tools to those seeking to optimize their fertility through the power of nutrition.

CHAPTER 2

UNDERSTANDING FERTILITY NUTRITION

Fertility nutrition is a nuanced realm that involves tailoring dietary choices to support reproductive health. It encompasses a strategic approach to nourishment, acknowledging the profound impact of specific nutrients on the intricate processes of conception and pregnancy.

Key aspects of understanding fertility nutrition include:

1. **Essential Nutrients:** Identifying and incorporating crucial nutrients like folic acid, iron, omega-3 fatty acids, and antioxidants that play pivotal roles in reproductive function.

2. **Hormonal Balance:** Recognizing the influence of diet on hormonal levels, aiming for a balanced endocrine system crucial for menstrual regularity and ovulation.

3. **Inflammation and Fertility:**
Understanding the connection between chronic inflammation and fertility challenges, and adopting an anti-inflammatory diet to mitigate potential risks.

4. **Weight and Fertility:** Acknowledging the impact of body weight on fertility, with guidance on achieving a healthy weight through balanced nutrition.

5. **Gut Health:** Exploring the link between gut microbiota and fertility, emphasizing the importance of a gut-friendly diet for overall reproductive wellness.

By delving into these aspects, individuals can gain a deeper appreciation for the profound role nutrition plays in optimizing fertility and laying a strong foundation for a healthy reproductive journey.

KEY NUTRIENTS FOR REPRODUCTIVE HEALTH

1. **Folic Acid:** Essential for proper neural tube development in early pregnancy, found in leafy greens, legumes, and fortified cereals.

2. **Iron:** Supports oxygen transport in the blood and prevents anemia, sourced from lean meats, beans, and fortified grains.

3. **Omega-3 Fatty Acids:** Critical for brain and eye development, abundant in fatty fish, flaxseeds, and walnuts.

4. **Calcium:** Vital for bone health, found in dairy products, fortified plant-based milks, and leafy greens.

5. **Vitamin D:** Aids in calcium absorption and plays a role in reproductive hormone regulation; sunlight, fatty fish, and fortified foods are sources.

6. **Vitamin C:** Boosts iron absorption, present in citrus fruits, strawberries, and bell peppers.

7. **Zinc:** Important for immune function and fertility, sources include meat, dairy, and nuts.

8. **Antioxidants:** Found in fruits and vegetables, they help combat oxidative stress and support overall reproductive health.

Ensuring a well-rounded diet that includes these nutrients is integral to promoting reproductive wellness and increasing the likelihood of a healthy pregnancy.

THE IMPACT OF DIET ON FERTILITY

Dietary choices exert a profound influence on fertility, affecting various aspects of reproductive health. Here are key ways in which diet impacts fertility:

1. **Hormonal Balance:** Nutrient-rich foods contribute to hormonal equilibrium, crucial for regular menstrual cycles and ovulation.

2. **Weight Management:** Maintaining a healthy weight through balanced nutrition positively influences fertility, preventing complications associated with both underweight and overweight conditions.

3. **Inflammation Reduction:** A diet rich in anti-inflammatory foods helps reduce chronic inflammation, lowering the risk of fertility-related issues.

4. **Insulin Sensitivity:** Balanced nutrition supports insulin sensitivity, playing a role in conditions like polycystic ovary syndrome (PCOS) that can affect fertility.

5. **Egg and Sperm Health:** Specific nutrients, such as antioxidants and omega-3 fatty acids, contribute to the health of eggs and sperm, impacting fertility at a cellular level.

6. **Nutrient Absorption:** Adequate intake of vitamins and minerals ensures proper nutrient absorption, supporting overall reproductive function.

Understanding these connections empowers individuals to make informed dietary choices, fostering an environment conducive to optimal fertility and increasing the chances of a successful conception.

CHAPTER 3

FOUNDATIONAL INGREDIENTS

Building a foundation for fertility-friendly meals involves incorporating key ingredients rich in essential nutrients. Here are some foundational ingredients to prioritize:

1. **Leafy Greens:** Spinach, kale, and Swiss chard provide a wealth of vitamins, minerals, and antioxidants crucial for reproductive health.

2. **Lean Proteins:** Opt for sources like poultry, fish, beans, and lentils to ensure a steady supply of protein without excessive saturated fats.

3. **Whole Grains:** Quinoa, brown rice, and oats offer complex carbohydrates, fiber, and essential nutrients vital for sustained energy and reproductive health.

4. **Healthy Fats:** Include sources of omega-3 fatty acids such as salmon, flaxseeds, and walnuts to support brain and hormonal health.

5. **Colorful Vegetables:** A variety of colorful vegetables ensures a diverse range of vitamins and minerals, contributing to overall well-being.

6. **Berries:** Packed with antioxidants, berries like blueberries and strawberries can combat oxidative stress and support reproductive function.

7. **Nuts and Seeds:** Almonds, chia seeds, and pumpkin seeds provide essential nutrients, including zinc and omega-3 fatty acids.

By incorporating these foundational ingredients into your meals, you lay the groundwork for a nutrient-dense diet that promotes reproductive wellness.

OVERVIEW OF FOODS RICH IN ESSENTIAL NUTRIENTS

1. **Folic Acid:**
   - Sources: Leafy greens (spinach, kale), lentils, fortified cereals, avocado.
   - Importance: Crucial for early fetal development and preventing neural tube defects.

2. **Iron:**
   - Sources: Lean meats (chicken, beef), beans, lentils, fortified grains.
   - Importance: Supports oxygen transport in the blood, preventing anemia.

3. **Omega-3 Fatty Acids:**
   - Sources: Fatty fish (salmon, mackerel),walnuts, flaxseeds.
   - Importance: Supports brain and eye development, reduces inflammation.

4. **Calcium:**
   - Sources: leafy greens, fortified plant-based milks, diary products.
   - Importance: Vital for bone health and muscle function.

5. **Vitamin D:**
   - Sources: Sunlight, fatty fish (salmon, tuna), fortified foods.
   - Importance: Aids in calcium absorption, regulates reproductive hormones.

6. **Vitamin C:**
   - Sources: Citrus fruits (oranges, and lemons), strawberries, and bell peppers.
   - Importance: Enhances iron absorption, supports immune function.

7. **Zinc:**
   - Sources: Meat, dairy, nuts, seeds.
   - Importance: Essential for immune function and fertility.

Incorporating a diverse range of these nutrient-rich foods into your diet provides a holistic approach to supporting reproductive health and fertility.

IMPORTANCE OF A BALANCED DIET

Maintaining a balanced diet is paramount for overall health and, specifically, for optimizing fertility. Here's why a balanced diet holds such significance:

1. **Optimal Nutrient Intake:** A balanced diet ensures the intake of a variety of nutrients necessary for reproductive health, including vitamins, minerals, proteins, and essential fatty acids.

2. **Hormonal Regulation:** Balanced nutrition contributes to hormonal balance, supporting regular menstrual cycles, ovulation, and overall reproductive function.

3. **Weight Management:** A balanced diet helps achieve and maintain a healthy weight, reducing the risk of fertility-related complications associated with both underweight and overweight conditions.

4. **Energy and Vitality:** Proper nutrition provides sustained energy levels, promoting overall well-being and vitality necessary for the demands of conception and pregnancy.

5. **Reduced Inflammation:** A balanced diet with anti-inflammatory properties helps mitigate chronic inflammation, decreasing the risk of fertility challenges linked to inflammatory conditions.

6. **Cellular Health:** Nutrient-rich foods support the health of eggs and sperm at a cellular level, enhancing the chances of successful conception.

By prioritizing a balanced and diverse range of foods, individuals create an environment conducive to reproductive wellness, laying a solid foundation for their fertility journey.

CHAPTER 4

BREAKFAST BOOSTERS

Start your day with fertility-friendly breakfast options designed to provide essential nutrients and sustained energy. Here are some breakfast ideas to kickstart your mornings:

1. **Fertility Smoothie:**
   - Blend spinach, berries, Greek yogurt, and a sprinkle of chia seeds for a nutrient-packed and delicious smoothie.

2. **Oatmeal Power Bowl:**
   - Top your oatmeal with sliced almonds, fresh fruits, and a drizzle of honey for a fiber-rich and nutrient-dense breakfast.

3. **Egg and Avocado Toast:**
   - Poached or scrambled eggs on whole-grain toast with avocado slices for a protein and healthy fat-rich breakfast.

4. **Quinoa Breakfast Bowl:**
   - Cooked quinoa with almond milk, topped with nuts, seeds, and diced fruits for a wholesome and protein-rich option.

5. **Greek Yogurt Parfait:**
   - Layer Greek yogurt with granola, berries, and a touch of honey for a balanced and satisfying breakfast.

6. **Salmon Bagel with Cream Cheese:**
   - Whole-grain bagel topped with smoked salmon, cream cheese, and fresh herbs for omega-3 fatty acids and protein.

Ensure your breakfast includes a mix of proteins, healthy fats, and complex carbohydrates to provide sustained energy and essential nutrients for reproductive health.

NUTRIENT–PACKED BREAKFAST RECIPES

Certainly! Here are two nutrient-packed breakfast recipes tailored to support reproductive health:

1. **Spinach and Berry Breakfast Smoothie**:

- Ingredients:

- 1 cup spinach leaves
- 1/2 cup mixed berries (strawberries, blueberries, raspberries)
- 1/2 banana
- 1/2 cup Greek yogurt
- 1 tablespoon chia seeds
- 1 cup almond milk
- Ice cubes (optional)

- Instructions:

1. Blend spinach, berries, banana, Greek yogurt, chia seeds, and almond milk until smooth.
2. Add ice cubes if needed and re-blend.
3. Pour into a glass and enjoy this nutrient-rich, fertility-boosting smoothie.

2. **Quinoa Breakfast Bowl with Nuts and Berries:

- Ingredients:

   - 1/2 cup cooked quinoa
   - 1/4 cup mixed nuts (walnuts and almond)
   - 1/2 cup mixed berries (blueberries, raspberries)
   - 1 tablespoon honey
   - 1/2 cup Greek yogurt

- Instructions:

   1. In a bowl, combine cooked quinoa, mixed nuts, and berries.
   2. Drizzle honey over the mixture and top with Greek yogurt.
   3. Gently mix and savor this nutrient-packed and protein-rich breakfast bowl.

These recipes not only provide essential nutrients but also offer a delightful start to your day with flavors that support reproductive wellness.

BENEFITS OF STARTING THE DAY WITH FERTILITY-FRIENDLY FOODS

1. **Optimized Nutrient Intake:** Beginning your day with fertility-friendly foods ensures an early intake of essential nutrients crucial for reproductive health, including vitamins, minerals, and antioxidants.

2. **Steady Energy Levels:** Nutrient-dense breakfasts, rich in complex carbohydrates and proteins, provide sustained energy throughout the morning, supporting overall well-being and vitality.

3. **Hormonal Balance:** Fertility-friendly breakfasts contribute to hormonal equilibrium, fostering regular menstrual cycles and optimal reproductive function.

4. **Improved Insulin Sensitivity:** Choosing foods that promote stable blood sugar levels helps maintain insulin sensitivity, positively impacting conditions like polycystic ovary syndrome (PCOS).

5. **Enhanced Metabolism:** A well-balanced breakfast kickstarts your metabolism, aiding in weight management, a crucial factor for fertility.

6. **Reduced Inflammation:** Including anti-inflammatory foods in your morning routine helps mitigate chronic inflammation, lowering the risk of fertility challenges associated with inflammatory conditions.

7. **Cellular Support:** Nutrient-packed breakfasts provide support at a cellular level, promoting the health of eggs and sperm and increasing the likelihood of successful conception.

By prioritizing fertility-friendly foods in the morning, you set a positive tone for the day, nurturing your reproductive health and laying the foundation for a successful fertility journey.

CHAPTER 5

LUNCHTIME NOURISHMENT

Elevate your midday meal with fertility-nourishing lunch options. Here are some ideas to ensure your lunch supports reproductive health:

1. **Grilled Chicken Salad:**
   - Ingredients: Grilled chicken breast, mixed greens, cherry tomatoes, cucumber, and a sprinkle of pumpkin seeds. Dress with olive oil and lemon.

2. **Quinoa and Vegetable Stir-Fry:**
   - Ingredients: Quinoa, assorted colorful vegetables (bell peppers, broccoli, carrots), tofu or shrimp, and a light soy-ginger dressing.

3. **Salmon and Avocado Wrap:**
   - Ingredients: Whole-grain wrap filled with grilled salmon, avocado slices, leafy greens, and a yogurt-based sauce.

4. **Mediterranean Chickpea Bowl:**
   - Ingredients: Chickpeas, cherry tomatoes, cucumber, olives, feta cheese, and a drizzle of olive oil. Serve over a bed of spinach or quinoa.

5. **Sweet Potato and Black Bean Salad:**
   - Ingredients: Roasted sweet potato cubes, black beans, corn, red onion, and cilantro. Toss with lime vinaigrette.

6. **Vegetable and Lentil Soup:**
   - Ingredients: Lentils, assorted vegetables (carrots, celery, spinach), vegetable broth, and spices. A hearty, nutrient-rich soup option.

Ensure your lunch includes a mix of lean proteins, whole grains, and colorful vegetables to maintain energy levels and provide the necessary nutrients for reproductive health.

RECIPES FOCUSING ON FERTILITY-BOOSTING INGREDIENTS FOR LUNCH

1. **Quinoa and Salmon Power Bowl:**

- Ingredients:

- 1 cup cooked quinoa
- Grilled or baked salmon fillet
- Steamed broccoli and carrots
- Avocado slices
- Lemon-tahini dressing

- Instructions:

1. Arrange quinoa as the base in a bowl.
2. Top with grilled salmon, steamed veggies, and avocado slices.
3. Drizzle with lemon-tahini dressing for a nutrient-packed lunch.

2. **Chickpea and Spinach Stuffed Bell Peppers:**

- Ingredients:

- Bell peppers, halved and cleaned
- Chickpeas, cooked
- Sautéed spinach and red onion
- Feta cheese
- Mediterranean spices

- Instructions:

1. Mix chickpeas, sautéed spinach, red onion, and feta cheese.
2. Stuff the mixture into halved bell peppers.
3. Bake until peppers are tender for a fertility-boosting lunch.

3. **Shrimp and Avocado Salad:**

- Ingredients:

- Grilled shrimp
- Mixed greens
- Cherry tomatoes
- Avocado slices
- Balsamic vinaigrette

- Instructions:

   1. Toss grilled shrimp, mixed greens, cherry tomatoes, and avocado slices.
   2. Drizzle with balsamic vinaigrette for a refreshing and fertility-friendly salad.

These recipes not only offer delicious flavors but also incorporate fertility-enhancing ingredients to support reproductive health during lunchtime.

TIPS FOR CREATING BALANCED MEALS

1. **Incorporate a Variety of Food Groups:**
   - Include a mix of lean proteins, whole grains, fruits, vegetables, and healthy fats in each meal for a well-rounded nutritional profile.

2. **Colorful Plate:**
   - Aim for a colorful meal by including a range of fruits and veggies. Different colors often indicate diverse nutrients.

3. **Portion Control:**
   - Be mindful of portion sizes to prevent overeating. Use smaller plates to help control portions and avoid unnecessary calorie intake.

4. **Protein-Packed Choices:**
   - Include lean protein sources like poultry, fish, tofu, beans, and nuts to support muscle health and keep you feeling full.

5. **Whole Grains:**
   - Opt for whole grains like brown rice, quinoa, and whole wheat bread to provide complex carbohydrates and fiber for sustained energy.

6. **Healthy Fats:**
   - Include sources of healthy fats such as avocados, nuts, and olive oil to support brain health and absorb fat-soluble vitamins.

7. **Mindful Cooking Methods:
   - Choose healthier cooking methods like grilling, baking, steaming, or sautéing instead of deep-frying to retain nutrients.

8. **Hydration:**
   - Drink water with each meal to stay
hydrated. Avoid sugary drinks and excessive
coffee consumption.

9. **Balance Over Time:**
   - Achieve balance over the course of the day
if a single meal doesn't cover all food groups.
Your overall daily intake matters.

10. **Listen to Your Body:**
   - Pay attention to hunger and fullness cues.
Eat when hungry, and stop when satisfied to
avoid overeating.

By integrating these tips, you can create meals
that not only taste good but also provide the
necessary nutrients for overall health and
fertility support.

CHAPTER 6

DINNER DELIGHTS

Wrap up your day with nourishing and fertility-friendly dinner options. Here are some delightful recipes to consider:

1. **Salmon and Asparagus Foil Packets:**

- **Ingredients**:

- Salmon fillet
- Asparagus spears
- Lemon slices
- Garlic, minced
- Olive oil
- Fresh dill

- **Instructions**:

1. Place salmon and asparagus on a foil sheet.
2. Drizzle with olive oil, add minced garlic, lemon slices, and fresh dill.
3. Seal the foil packet and bake for a flavorful and nutritious dinner.

2. **Vegetarian Lentil Stew:**

   - **Ingredients**:

    - Lentils
    - Tomatoes, diced
    - Carrots, diced
    - Spinach
    - Vegetable broth
    - Cumin, coriander, and paprika for
seasoning

   - **Instructions**:

    1. Cook lentils in vegetable broth with diced
tomatoes and carrots.
    2. Add spinach and season with cumin,
coriander, and paprika for a hearty stew.

3. **Turkey and Sweet Potato Skillet:**

   - **Ingredients**:

    - Ground turkey
    - Sweet potatoes, diced
    - Bell peppers, diced
    - Onion, diced
    - Garlic, minced
    - Cumin and chili powder for seasoning

- Instructions:

    1. Cook ground turkey with sweet potatoes, bell peppers, onion, and garlic.

    2. Season with cumin and chili powder for a tasty and protein-packed skillet.

These dinner delights not only provide a satisfying end to your day but also offer essential nutrients to support reproductive health.

DINNER RECIPES DESIGNED FOR REPRODUCTIVE HEALTH

1. **Quinoa-Stuffed Bell Peppers:**

- Ingredients:

- Bell peppers, halved
- Quinoa, cooked
- Black beans, corn, diced tomatoes
- Cumin, paprika, and garlic powder for seasoning
- Shredded cheese (optional)

- **Instructions**:

    1. Mix cooked quinoa with black beans, corn, and diced tomatoes.
    2. Season with cumin, paprika, and garlic powder.
    3. Stuff bell peppers with the mixture and bake until peppers are tender.
    4. Optionally, top with shredded cheese.

2. **Mediterranean Baked Chicken:**

- **Ingredients**:

    - Chicken breasts
    - Cherry tomatoes, olives, and artichoke hearts
    - Olive oil, garlic, oregano, and lemon juice for seasoning

- **Instructions**:

    1. Place chicken breasts in a baking dish.
    2. Surround with cherry tomatoes, olives, and artichoke hearts.
    3. Drizzle with olive oil, garlic, oregano, and lemon juice.
    4. Bake until chicken is cooked through.

3. **Vegetable Stir-Fry with Tofu:**

- Ingredients:

- Tofu, cubed
- Broccoli, bell peppers, carrots
- Ginger, garlic, and soy sauce for seasoning
- Brown rice, cooked

- Instructions:

1. Sauté tofu with broccoli, bell peppers, and carrots.
2. Add ginger, garlic, and soy sauce for flavor.
3. Serve over cooked brown rice for a balanced and fertility-friendly stir-fry.

These recipes not only prioritize reproductive health but also offer delicious and wholesome options for a nutritious dinner.

INCORPORATING VARIETY AND FLAVORS

Enhance your meals with a diverse range of ingredients, textures, and flavors to make your diet more enjoyable and nutrient-rich. Here's how to incorporate variety and flavors into your meals:

1. **Explore Global Cuisines:**
   - Try recipes from different cultures to introduce a variety of herbs, spices, and cooking techniques.

2. **Colorful Produce:**
   - Include a spectrum of colorful fruits and vegetables to ensure a diverse range of nutrients and antioxidants.

3. **Experiment with Herbs and Spices:**
   - Use fresh herbs like basil, cilantro, or mint, and experiment with spices to add depth and flavor to your dishes.

4. **Mix Proteins:**
   - Combine different protein sources, such as poultry, fish, tofu, or legumes, to diversify amino acid profiles.

5. **Grains Galore:**
   - Explore a variety of whole grains like quinoa, farro, and barley for unique textures and nutritional benefits.

6. **Creative Salads:**
   - Build salads with a mix of leafy greens, nuts, seeds, fruits, and a variety of colorful vegetables for both taste and nutrition.

7. **Play with Textures:**
   - Incorporate a mix of crunchy, chewy, and tender textures in your meals to make them more interesting.

8. **Savory and Sweet Combinations:**
   - Experiment with dishes that combine savory and sweet elements to stimulate your taste buds.

9. **Homemade Sauces and Dressings:**
   - Create your own sauces and dressings using a variety of herbs, spices, and healthy oils for added flavor.

10. **Seasonal Eating:**
   - Embrace seasonal produce to enjoy the freshest flavors and nutritional benefits.

By embracing variety and experimenting with flavors, you not only make your meals more exciting but also ensure a broader spectrum of nutrients, contributing to a well-rounded and fertility-friendly diet.

CHAPTER 7

SNACKS FOR FERTILITY

Keep your energy levels stable and support reproductive health with these nutritious and fertility-friendly snack ideas:

1. **Greek Yogurt with Berries:**
   - Combine Greek yogurt with fresh berries for a protein-packed and antioxidant-rich snack.

2. **Almond Butter and Banana Slices:**
   - Spread almond butter on banana slices for a satisfying combination of healthy fats, protein, and natural sweetness.

3. **Vegetable Sticks with Hummus:**
   - Enjoy a crunchy snack by dipping carrot, cucumber, and bell pepper sticks into hummus for a nutrient boost.

4. **Hard-Boiled Eggs:**
   - Hard-boil eggs in advance for a convenient and protein-rich snack.

5. **Trail Mix:**
   - Create a custom trail mix with a mix of nuts, seeds, and dried fruits for a balanced blend of nutrients.

6. **Cottage Cheese with Pineapple:**
   - Pair cottage cheese with fresh pineapple chunks for a calcium-rich and tasty snack.

7. **Chia Pudding:**
   - Make chia pudding with almond milk and top it with berries for a satisfying and omega-3 rich snack.

8. **Whole Grain Crackers with Avocado:**
   - Spread avocado on whole grain crackers for a combination of healthy fats and fiber.

9. **Oatmeal Energy Bites:**
   - Mix oats, nut butter, honey, and dark chocolate chips to create energy bites for a quick and tasty snack.

10. **Edamame Pods:**
   - Enjoy edamame pods sprinkled with sea salt for a protein-packed and satisfying snack.

Incorporating these snacks into your day can contribute to a well-balanced diet, providing the nutrients necessary for optimal reproductive health.

HEALTHY SNACK IDEAS BETWEEN MEALS

Certainly! Here are some healthy snack ideas to keep you energized between meals:

1. **Apple Slices with Nut Butter:**
   - Pair apple slices with almond or peanut butter for a satisfying combination of fiber and healthy fats.

2. **Yogurt Parfait:**
   - Layer Greek yogurt with granola and fresh berries for a protein-rich and flavorful snack.

3. **Mixed Nuts and Dried Fruits:**
   - Create your own trail mix with a mix of nuts (almonds, walnuts) and dried fruits (apricots, cranberries).

4. **Hummus and Veggie Sticks:**
   - Dip cucumber, carrot, and bell pepper sticks into hummus for a crunchy and nutrient-packed snack.

5. **Hard-Boiled Eggs with Cherry Tomatoes:**
   - Pair hard-boiled eggs with cherry tomatoes for a protein-rich and convenient snack.

6. **Cottage Cheese with Pineapple:**
   - Combine cottage cheese with fresh pineapple chunks for a refreshing and calcium-rich option.

7. **Greek Yogurt Bark:**
   - Mix Greek yogurt with honey and freeze for a delicious and satisfying yogurt bark.

8. **Chia Seed Pudding:**
   - Make chia seed pudding with almond milk and top it with sliced strawberries or blueberries.

9. **Whole Grain Crackers with Cheese:**
   - Enjoy whole grain crackers with a small portion of your favorite cheese for a balanced and tasty snack.

10. **Roasted Chickpeas:**
    - Season chickpeas with spices and roast them for a crunchy and protein-packed snack.

These snacks provide a mix of nutrients, helping to curb hunger and maintain energy levels between meals.

PORTABLE SNACK OPTIONS FOR BUSY LIFESTYLES

For those on the go, here are some convenient and portable snack options to keep you fueled throughout your busy day:

1. **Nut and Seed Bars:**
   - Choose bars made with nuts, seeds, and dried fruits for a portable and energy-boosting snack.

2. **Fresh Fruit**:**
   - Grab fruits like apples, bananas, or oranges for a quick and easily transportable snack.

3. **String Cheese**:**
   - Single-serving string cheese provides protein and calcium in a convenient, grab-and-go form.

4. **Individual Nut Packs:**
   - Pre-portioned nut packs with almonds, walnuts, or mixed nuts offer a portable source of healthy fats and protein.

5. **Greek Yogurt Cups:**
   - Opt for individual-sized Greek yogurt cups with a spoon for a protein-rich and convenient snack.

6. **Whole Grain Crackers with Hummus Cups:**
   - Pack whole grain crackers with individual hummus cups for a satisfying and portable combo.

7. **Baby Carrots with Guacamole:**
   - Pre-cut baby carrots with small containers of guacamole provide a nutrient-packed and portable snack.

8. **Dried Seaweed Snacks:**
   - Crispy dried seaweed snacks are low in calories and can be easily carried in your bag.

9. **Trail Mix Packs:**
   - Purchase pre-packaged trail mix with nuts, seeds, and dried fruits for a quick and portable energy boost.

10. **Protein Bars:**
   - Select protein bars with minimal added sugars and a good balance of protein and fiber for a convenient snack.

These options are not only portable but also offer a mix of nutrients to keep you fueled and satisfied during your busy schedule.

CHAPTER 8

BEVERAGES THAT SUPPORT FERTILITY

Stay hydrated with beverages that contribute to reproductive health. Consider incorporating these fertility-friendly drinks into your routine:

1. **Green Tea:**
   - Rich in antioxidants, green tea may support fertility by reducing oxidative stress. Limit caffeine intake for optimal benefits.

2. **Herbal Teas:**
   - Choose caffeine-free herbal teas like peppermint, chamomile, or red raspberry leaf for a soothing and hydrating option.

3. **Water with Lemon:**
   - Plain water infused with lemon provides hydration while offering a refreshing and low-calorie option.

4. **Fruit-infused Water:**
   - Infuse water with slices of fruits like berries, citrus, or cucumber for a flavorful and hydrating choice.

5. **Pomegranate Juice:**
   - Pomegranate juice is rich in antioxidants and may have positive effects on reproductive health. Opt for pure, unsweetened juice.

6. **Milk or Plant-Based Milk:**
   - Dairy or fortified plant-based milk provides calcium and vitamin D, essential for bone health and hormonal balance.

7. **Smoothies:**
   - Blend fertility-friendly ingredients like berries, spinach, Greek yogurt, and a splash of almond milk for a nutrient-packed beverage.

8. **Coconut Water:**
   - Natural coconut water is a hydrating option that provides electrolytes without added sugars.

9. **Ginger Tea:**
   - Ginger tea may have anti-inflammatory properties and can be a warming and soothing beverage.

10. **Watermelon Juice:**
   - Watermelon is hydrating and contains lycopene, which may have benefits for fertility. Blend fresh watermelon for a refreshing drink.

Remember to balance your beverage choices with overall hydration needs and maintain a healthy lifestyle for optimal reproductive well-being.

DRINKS THAT CONTRIBUTE TO REPRODUCTIVE WELL-BEING

Incorporate these beverages into your routine to support reproductive health and overall well-being:

1. **Fertility Smoothies:**
   - Blend fruits like berries, banana, and spinach with Greek yogurt and a splash of almond milk for a nutrient-packed smoothie.

2. **Green Tea:**
   - Green tea, rich in antioxidants, may have positive effects on fertility by reducing oxidative stress.

3. **Pomegranate Juice:**
   - Pomegranate juice contains antioxidants and has been associated with potential benefits for reproductive health.

4. **Herbal Teas:**
   - Choose fertility-friendly herbal teas like red raspberry leaf, peppermint, or chamomile for their soothing properties.

5. **Water with Lemon:**
   - Stay hydrated with plain water infused with fresh lemon, providing a refreshing and low-calorie option.

6. **Milk or Fortified Plant-Based Milk:**
   - Dairy or plant-based milk options contribute to calcium and vitamin D intake, essential for reproductive health.

7. **Beetroot Juice:**
   - Beetroot juice is rich in nitrates and antioxidants, potentially supporting blood flow and overall cardiovascular health.

8. **Turmeric Golden Milk:**
   - Mix turmeric with warm milk and a dash of honey for a soothing and anti-inflammatory beverage.

9. **Berry-Infused Water:**
   - Enhance your hydration with water infused with berries, providing a subtle flavor and antioxidants.

10. **Coconut Water:**
   - Natural coconut water is hydrating and provides electrolytes without added sugars.

Incorporating these drinks into your diet can contribute to a well-rounded approach to reproductive well-being. As always, it's essential to maintain a balanced and healthy lifestyle for overall health benefits.

IMPORTANCE OF HYDRATION

Staying adequately hydrated is crucial for overall health, and it plays a significant role in supporting reproductive well-being. Here's why hydration is important:

1. **Optimal Body Function:**
   - Hydration is essential for proper functioning of bodily systems, including the reproductive system. It helps maintain fluid balance and supports various physiological processes.

2. **Cervical Mucus Production:**
   - Well-hydrated individuals tend to have better-quality cervical mucus. Proper cervical mucus is important for sperm transport and fertility.

3. **Uterine Health:**
   - Adequate hydration contributes to uterine health by ensuring a well-lubricated environment, potentially supporting embryo implantation.

4. **Blood Flow and Circulation:**

   - Hydration is crucial for maintaining proper blood viscosity, facilitating nutrient and oxygen transport to reproductive organs.

5. **Sperm Health:**

   - For men, staying hydrated is linked to better sperm health. Dehydration can lead to decreased semen volume and concentration.

6. **Hormonal Balance:**

   - Proper hydration supports hormonal balance, which is essential for regular menstrual cycles and overall reproductive function.

7. **Preventing UTIs:**

   - Hydration helps prevent urinary tract infections (UTIs), which can negatively impact reproductive health.

8. **Temperature Regulation:**

   - Adequate water intake helps regulate body temperature, preventing overheating, especially in situations that may affect fertility.

9. **Toxin Elimination:**
   - Hydration supports the elimination of waste and toxins from the body, promoting a healthier internal environment.

10. **General Well-being:**
   - Staying hydrated contributes to overall well-being, reducing fatigue and promoting energy levels necessary for a healthy reproductive journey.

Remember to drink water consistently throughout the day to maintain proper hydration.

CHAPTER 9

MEAL PLANNING AND PREPARATION TIPS

Efficient meal planning and preparation can make it easier to maintain a balanced and fertility-friendly diet. The following tips can help to streamline the process

1. **Create a Weekly Menu:**
   - Plan your meals for the week, incorporating a variety of nutrients and fertility-friendly ingredients.

2. **Include a Mix of Food Groups:**
   - Ensure each meal includes a balance of lean proteins, whole grains, fruits, vegetables, and healthy fats for comprehensive nutrition.

3. **Batch Cooking:**
   - Cook in batches and prepare larger quantities of staple foods that can be portioned and stored for later use. This saves time on busy days.

4. **Prep Ingredients in Advance:**
   - Wash, chop, and prep vegetables, fruits, and proteins ahead of time to streamline cooking during the week.

5. **Invest in Storage Containers:**
   - Have a variety of storage containers for portioning and storing meals. This makes it easy to grab a healthy option when needed.

6. **Keep Healthy Snacks Ready:**
   - Pre-portion snacks like nuts, fruits, and cut vegetables in easily accessible containers for quick and healthy snacking.

7. **Explore One-Pan Meals:**
   - Experiment with one-pan or sheet pan meals that simplify cooking and minimize cleanup.

8. **Plan for Leftovers:**
   - Embrace leftovers as a time-saving strategy. Cook extra portions that can be enjoyed the next day.

9. **Incorporate Freezer-Friendly Options:**
   - Prepare freezer-friendly meals for nights when you don't have time to cook. Casseroles, stews, and soups usually freeze well.

10. **Stay Flexible:**
   - Allow for flexibility in your meal plan. Life can be unpredictable, so having some go-to quick and healthy options is beneficial.

11. **Use a Grocery List:**
   - Create a detailed grocery list based on your meal plan to ensure you have all the necessary ingredients on hand.

12. **Explore New Recipes:**
   - Keep things interesting by trying out new fertility-friendly recipes. This adds variety and excitement to your meals.

By incorporating these meal planning and preparation tips, you can simplify your approach to eating healthily, saving time and ensuring you have nutritious options readily available.

PRACTICAL ADVICE FOR PLANNING FERTILITY-FOCUSED MEALS

When planning meals with a focus on fertility, consider these practical tips to support your reproductive health:

1. **prioritize nutrient-rich foods:**
   - Emphasize whole, nutrient-dense foods such as fruits, vegetables, lean proteins, whole grains, and healthy fats in your meals.

2. **Include Folate-Rich Foods:**
   - Incorporate folate-rich foods like leafy greens, legumes, and fortified grains to support early fetal development.

3. **Opt for Omega-3 Fatty Acids:**
   - Choose sources of omega-3 fatty acids such as fatty fish (salmon, mackerel), flaxseeds, and walnuts to support reproductive health.

4. **Ensure Adequate Iron Intake:**
   - Include iron-rich foods like lean meats, beans, and fortified cereals to prevent anemia and support overall health.

5. **Balance Protein Intake:**
   - Include a variety of protein sources such as poultry, fish, eggs, dairy, tofu, and legumes for a well-rounded amino acid profile.

6. **Choose Whole Grains:**
   - Opt for whole grains like brown rice, quinoa, and oats to provide complex carbohydrates and fiber.

7. **Incorporate Colorful Vegetables:**
   - Include a rainbow of vegetables to ensure a diverse range of antioxidants and phytonutrients.

8. **Stay Hydrated:**
   - Drink plenty of water throughout the day to maintain hydration, which is essential for reproductive health.

9. **Moderate Caffeine Intake:**
   - Limit caffeine intake and choose decaffeinated options when possible, as excessive caffeine may impact fertility.

10. **Limit Processed Foods:**
   - Minimize processed and sugary foods, focusing on whole, minimally processed options for optimal nutrition.

11. **Consider Herbal Infusions:**
   - Explore herbal infusions like red raspberry leaf tea, which is believed to support reproductive health.

12. **Monitor Portion Sizes:**
   - Pay attention to portion sizes to maintain a healthy weight, as both underweight and overweight conditions can affect fertility.

13. **Include Dairy or Fortified Plant-Based Milk:**
   - Ensure adequate calcium and vitamin D intake by including dairy or fortified plant-based milk in your diet.

14. **Practice Mindful Eating:**
   - Eat mindfully, paying attention to hunger and fullness cues, and savor the flavors of your meals.

By incorporating these practical tips into your meal planning, you can create a fertility-focused diet that supports your reproductive goals and overall well-being.

TIME–SAVING STRATEGIES FOR BUSY SCHEDULES

Maintaining a fertility-focused diet on a busy schedule can be challenging, but these time-saving strategies can help you stay on track:

1. **Meal Prep on Weekends:**
   - Use weekends to batch cook and prepare meals for the upcoming week. This saves time during busy weekdays.

2. **Freezer-Friendly Options:**
   - Prepare freezer-friendly meals like soups, stews, and casseroles in advance for quick and convenient dinners.

3. **One-Pan Meals:**
   - Opt for one-pan or sheet pan meals that minimize prep and cleanup time. Roast vegetables and proteins together for a simple yet nutritious option.

4. **Quick and Healthy Snacks:**
   - Keep pre-portioned healthy snacks, like nuts, cut veggies, and yogurt, readily available for easy grabbing during busy moments.

5. **Pre-Cut Vegetables and Fruits:**
   - Wash, cut, and portion vegetables and fruits in advance to save time when assembling meals or snacks.

6. **Utilize Crockpot or Instant Pot:**
   - Slow cookers and pressure cookers are excellent time-savers. Throw ingredients in the morning, and have a ready-to-eat meal by evening.

7. **Pre-Pack Lunches:**
   - Pre-pack lunches the night before, ensuring you have a balanced and fertility-focused meal ready to take with you.

8. **Plan Simple Breakfasts:**
   - Choose quick and nutritious breakfast options like overnight oats, smoothies, or yogurt parfaits for a hassle-free start to the day.

9. **Grocery Shopping Efficiency:**
   - Plan your grocery list in advance and organize it by store sections to streamline your shopping trip.

10. **Delegate or Share Cooking Responsibilities:**
   - If possible, share cooking responsibilities with family members or consider a meal-sharing arrangement with friends.

11. **Embrace Convenience:**
   - Utilize healthy convenience options like pre-washed salads, pre-cooked grains, and rotisserie chicken for quicker meal assembly.

12. **Multitasking Cooking:**
   - Maximize time by multitasking during cooking. For example, chop vegetables while waiting for water to boil.

13. **Cook in Bulk:**
   - Cook larger quantities of certain staples like rice, quinoa, or grilled chicken, and use them throughout the week in different meals.

14. **Set a Cooking Schedule:**
   - Allocate specific times for cooking in your schedule, treating it like any other important appointment.

By incorporating these time-saving strategies, you can maintain a fertility-focused diet even during hectic schedules, making it more manageable and sustainable.

CHAPTER 10

LIFESTYLE FACTORS FOR FERTILITY

In addition to a fertility-focused diet, several lifestyle factors can impact reproductive health. Consider the following aspects to support fertility:

1. **Maintain a Healthy Weight:**
   - Both being underweight and overweight might have an impact on fertility. Go for a healthy weight by combining a nutritious diet with frequent exercise.

2. **Regular Exercise:**
   - Engage in moderate and regular physical activity, such as walking, jogging, or yoga, to support overall health and fertility.

3. **Manage Stress Levels:**
   - Chronic stress can impact reproductive hormones. Practice stress-reduction techniques such as mindfulness, meditation and deep breathing.

4. **Adequate Sleep:**
   - Ensure you get sufficient and quality sleep, as irregular sleep patterns can disrupt hormonal balance and affect fertility.

5. **Limit Alcohol Consumption:**
   - Excessive alcohol intake can impair fertility. Limit alcohol consumption to moderate levels or avoid it altogether when trying to conceive.

6. **Quit Smoking:**
   - Smoking has been linked to reduced fertility in both men and women. Quitting smoking can improve reproductive health.

7. **Limit Caffeine Intake:**
   - High caffeine consumption has been linked to delayed conception. Limit caffeine consumption and opt for decaffeinated options.

8. **Avoid Exposure to Harmful Substances:**
   - Minimize exposure to environmental toxins, chemicals, and pollutants that may negatively impact fertility.

9. **Regular Menstrual Cycle Monitoring:**
   - Regularly monitor your menstrual cycle to understand your fertility window and increase the chances of conception.

10. **Preconception Health Check:**
   - Schedule a preconception health check with your healthcare provider to address any underlying health conditions that may impact fertility.

11. **Understand Your Menstrual Health:**
   - Be aware of any irregularities in your menstrual cycle, as they can be indicators of hormonal imbalances affecting fertility.

12. **Fertility Supplements:**
   - Consider taking prenatal vitamins or fertility supplements, particularly if there are specific nutrient deficiencies.

13. **Limit Exposure to Heat:**
   - Avoid prolonged exposure to high temperatures, such as hot tubs or saunas, which may affect sperm production.

14. **Open Communication:**
   - Maintain open and supportive communication with your partner. Discussing fertility goals and concerns can strengthen your relationship during the conception journey.

Remember, individual factors can vary, and consulting with a healthcare professional is crucial for personalized advice and guidance based on your specific health needs.

BEYOND NUTRITION: OTHER FACTORS INFLUENCING FERTILITY

While nutrition plays a significant role, various factors beyond diet can impact fertility. Consider these aspects for a holistic approach to reproductive health:

1. **Age:**
   - Age is a crucial factor, and fertility tends to decline with age, especially for women. It's essential to be mindful of biological clocks when planning for conception.

2. **Regular Menstrual Cycles:**
   - Regular and predictable menstrual cycles are indicative of hormonal balance and overall reproductive health.

3. **Body Mass Index (BMI):**
   - Both low and high BMI can affect fertility. Maintaining a healthy weight contributes to hormonal balance and reproductive well-being.

4. **Underlying Health Conditions:**
   - Thyroid issues, endometriosis, and polycystic ovarian syndrome (PCOS) are a few diseases that might affect fertility. Addressing these conditions is crucial.

5. **Sexual Health:**
   - Address any concerns related to sexual health, including sexually transmitted infections (STIs), as they can affect fertility.

6. **Environmental Factors:**
   - Exposure to environmental toxins, pollutants, and certain chemicals can impact fertility. Minimize exposure where possible.

7. **Lifestyle Habits:**
   - Unhealthy lifestyle habits such as excessive alcohol intake, smoking, and drug use can negatively influence fertility.

8. **Stress Levels:**
   - Chronic stress can affect hormonal balance and disrupt the menstrual cycle. Stress management is essential for reproductive health.

9. **Sleep Patterns:**
   - Irregular sleep patterns or inadequate sleep can disrupt hormonal cycles and impact fertility.

10. **Medication and Supplements:**
   - Certain medications and supplements may affect fertility. Consult with a healthcare provider to assess the impact of any medications on reproductive health.

11. **Pelvic Inflammatory Disease (PID):**
   - Infections, particularly pelvic inflammatory disease, can lead to scarring and damage to reproductive organs, affecting fertility.

12. **Male Factors:**
   - Male fertility is equally important. Factors like sperm count, motility, and morphology can impact conception.

13. **Timing of Intercourse:**
   - Understanding the menstrual cycle and identifying the fertile window can optimize the chances of conception.

14. **Genetic Factors:**
   - Genetic factors can play a role in fertility. Consultation with a genetic counselor may be beneficial in certain cases.

15. **Medical Treatments:**
   - Previous medical treatments or surgeries may impact fertility. Talk to a healthcare professional about any medical history you may have.

Considering these factors alongside a nutritious diet provides a comprehensive approach to promoting fertility and increasing the likelihood of a healthy conception. Consulting with healthcare professionals can offer personalized guidance based on individual circumstances.

TIPS FOR MAINTAINING A HEALTHY LIFESTYLE

Maintaining a healthy lifestyle is essential for overall well-being, including reproductive health. Here are tips to help you lead a healthy and balanced life:

1. **Balanced Diet:**
   - Consume a variety of nutrient-dense foods, including fruits, vegetables, whole grains, lean meats, and healthy fats.

2. **Regular Exercise:**
   - Engage in regular physical activity, incorporating both aerobic exercises (e.g., walking, jogging) and strength training for overall fitness.

3. **Adequate Sleep:**
   - Prioritize good sleep hygiene and aim for 7-9 hours of quality sleep each night to support physical and mental well-being.

4. **Stress Management:**
   - Practice stress-reducing activities such as meditation, deep breathing, yoga, or mindfulness to manage stress effectively.

5. **Hydration:**
   - Stay well-hydrated by drinking plenty of water throughout the day to support bodily functions and overall health.

6. **Limit Alcohol Intake:**
   - If you drink alcohol, do so in moderation. For women, this generally means up to one drink per day.

7. **Quit Smoking:**
   - Quit smoking to improve overall health and reduce the risk of fertility-related complications.

8. **Mindful Eating:**
   - Practice mindful eating by paying attention to hunger and fullness cues, and savoring the flavors of your meals.

9. **Maintain a Healthy Weight:**
   - Combine a well-balanced diet with regular exercise to reach and maintain a healthy weight.

10. **Regular Health Check-ups:**
   - Schedule regular health check-ups and screenings to monitor your overall health and address any potential issues proactively.

11. **Limit Processed Foods:**
   - Minimize the intake of processed and sugary foods, opting for whole, unprocessed options whenever possible.

12. **Build Supportive Relationships:**
   - Cultivate strong social connections and build supportive relationships with family and friends for emotional well-being.

13. **Practice Safe Sex:**
   - If sexually active, practice safe sex to protect against sexually transmitted infections and promote reproductive health.

14. **Limit Screen Time:**
   - Reduce excessive screen time and allocate time for outdoor activities and face-to-face interactions.

15. **Stay Informed:**
   - Stay informed about your health, understand your family medical history, and communicate openly with healthcare providers.

16. **Self-Care Practices:**
   - Prioritize self-care practices such as taking breaks, enjoying hobbies, and incorporating activities that bring joy and relaxation.

17. **Limit Caffeine Intake:**
   - Moderate caffeine intake and choose decaffeinated options, especially if planning for conception.

18. **Set Realistic Goals:**
   - Set realistic and achievable health goals that align with your lifestyle and values.

Adopting these tips into your daily routine can contribute to a healthy lifestyle, supporting not only reproductive health but overall well-being. Remember that small, sustainable changes over time can lead to lasting benefits.

CONCLUSION

In conclusion, prioritizing a fertility-friendly lifestyle involves a holistic approach that goes beyond nutrition. Understanding and addressing various factors, from overall health to lifestyle habits, plays a crucial role in supporting reproductive well-being.

Recap of Key Points:

1. **Nutrient-Rich Diet:** Prioritize a diet rich in essential nutrients, including folate, omega-3 fatty acids, and antioxidants, to support reproductive health.

2. **Lifestyle Factors:** Beyond nutrition, factors such as maintaining a healthy weight, regular exercise, stress management, and avoiding harmful substances contribute to fertility.

3. **Environmental Considerations:** Limit exposure to environmental toxins and pollutants to create a healthier environment for conception.

4. **Healthy Habits:** Incorporate habits like adequate sleep, staying hydrated, and practicing safe sex to promote overall health.

5. **Regular Check-ups:** Schedule regular health check-ups and consultations with healthcare professionals to monitor and address any reproductive health concerns.

ENCOURAGEMENT FOR EMBRACING A FERTILITY-FRIENDLY DIET

Embracing a fertility-friendly diet is a positive and empowering step toward achieving reproductive goals. By making mindful food choices, incorporating nutrient-rich recipes, and adopting a healthy lifestyle, you are laying the foundation for a healthier and potentially more successful conception journey.

Remember, every individual's journey is unique. Be patient, stay informed, and seek guidance from healthcare professionals for personalized advice. Celebrate the small victories and progress along the way, and trust in the positive impact that a well-rounded, fertility-focused approach can have on your overall well-being.

Here's to your health, well-being, and the exciting possibilities that the journey toward fertility brings. Wishing you the best on your path to a healthy and fulfilling life.